VEGAN ANTI-INFLAMMATORY DIET COOKBOOK FOR SENIORS

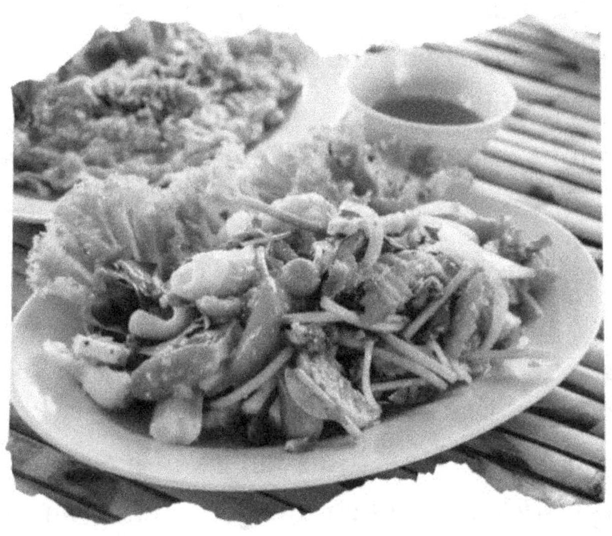

Quick and Easy Meal Prep Centered Around Foods To Fight Against Inflammation

KEVIN S. MAXWELL

EMAIL ME!

I know that exploring topics that involve food and nutrition can often lead to questions and uncertainty. I invite you to contact me with any questions you may have. I'm here to assist.

Please contact me through email at kevinmaxwelldiet@gmail.com, and I will try my best to respond to you within 24 hours.

Additionally, if you are interested in exploring other collections of my books. You can check out additional collections of my books by scanning the QR Code that is provided below.

HOW TO USE THIS COOKBOOK

Familiarize Yourself with the Cookbook:
Start by reading through the Vegan Anti-Inflammatory Diet Cookbook for Seniors. Familiarize yourself with the introduction, guidelines, and any tips provided by the author. Understand the structure of the cookbook, including the table of contents and recipe categories.

Plan Your Meals:
Take a moment to plan your meals using the cookbook. Choose recipes that appeal to your taste preferences and align with your nutritional goals. Consider creating a weekly or monthly meal plan to streamline your grocery shopping and meal preparation.

Create a Shopping List:
Based on the chosen recipes, create a shopping list of the required ingredients. Check your pantry and fridge for items you already have. This helps you organize your

shopping trip and ensures you have everything needed for your chosen recipes.

Batch Cooking and Meal Prep:
Simplify your daily routine by engaging in batch cooking and meal preparation. Prepare ingredients that can be used across multiple recipes, making it easier to assemble meals during the week. This proactive approach saves time and encourages adherence to the anti-inflammatory diet.

Enjoy and Adapt:
Begin incorporating the cookbook's recipes into your daily meals. Enjoy the flavors and benefits of plant-based, anti-inflammatory ingredients. Feel free to adapt recipes based on personal preferences and dietary needs. Regularly revisit the cookbook for variety, discover new favorites, and make this anti-inflammatory lifestyle an enjoyable and sustainable part of your routine.

TABLE OF CONTENT

Chickpea and Kale Salad

Sweet Potato and Lentil Buddha Bowl

Mediterranean Chickpea Salad

Teriyaki Tofu Stir-Fry

Roasted Vegetable Wrap

Cauliflower and Chickpea Tacos

Butternut Squash and Kale Risotto

DINNER

Lentil and Vegetable Stew

Chickpea and Spinach Curry

Quinoa-Stuffed Bell Peppers

Eggplant and Chickpea Tagine

Butternut Squash and Coconut Curry

Mediterranean Quinoa Salad

Vegan Buddha Bowl

Vegan Lentil and Vegetable Stir-Fry

Spaghetti Aglio e Olio with Roasted Vegetables

DESSERT

Chocolate Avocado Mousse

Vegan Berry Parfait

Peanut Butter Banana Ice Cream

Coconut Bliss Balls

Mango Sorbet

Oatmeal Raisin Cookies

Vegan Chocolate Chip Banana Bread

Raspberry Chia Seed Pudding

Almond Butter Energy Bites

Apple Cinnamon Baked Oatmeal

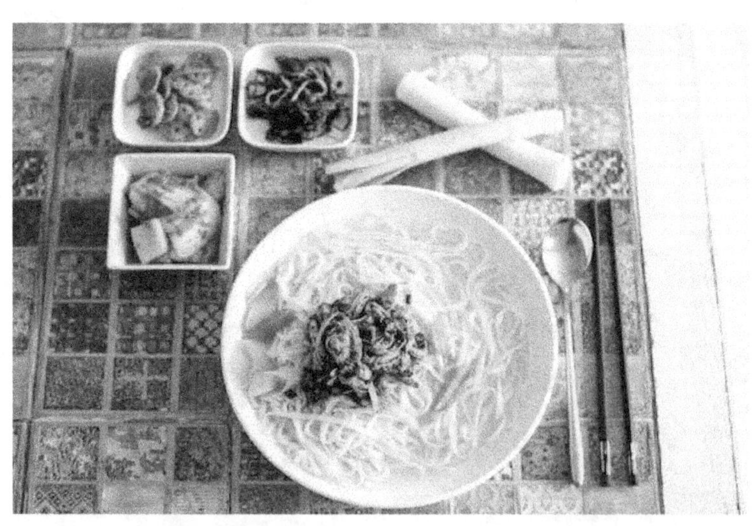

INTRODUCTION

Meet Harold. At 78, Harold was known for his gentle demeanor and a twinkle in his eye that hinted at a lifetime of wisdom. However, he faced a daily battle with inflammation, aches, and pains that often made simple tasks seem Herculean.

Harold had tried various medications over the years, but the side effects were a constant reminder of their limitations. One day, as he perused the shelves of the local bookstore, a colorful cookbook caught his eye – "Vegan Anti-Inflammatory Diet Cookbook For Seniors." Intrigued, he decided to give it a try.

The cookbook, penned by a nutritionist named Dr. Emily Turner, promised a holistic approach to managing inflammation through plant-based recipes. With hope in his heart, Harold started experimenting with the delicious and nutrient-packed meals within its pages.

His kitchen soon became a haven of vibrant colors and rich aromas. Harold discovered the joy of cooking with fresh vegetables, legumes, and whole grains. The recipes not only appealed to his taste buds but also seemed to work wonders on his inflammation. He felt lighter, more energetic, and the persistent aches began to subside.

As the weeks went by, Harold's newfound culinary adventure turned into a passion. He began sharing his plant-based creations with friends and neighbors, many of whom were surprised by the flavorful and satisfying nature of vegan cuisine. Soon, a small community of seniors formed, all inspired by Harold's journey and the healing power of a vegan anti-inflammatory diet.

Harold's story spread beyond the town, reaching the ears of Dr. Emily Turner herself. Intrigued by his success, she decided to visit the town to meet Harold and learn more about his experiences. The meeting was filled with laughter, shared meals, and a profound connection between a wise old man and a passionate nutritionist.

Together, they collaborated to create a follow-up cookbook, incorporating Harold's favorite recipes and personal tips. The "Harold's Healing Kitchen" cookbook became a bestseller, helping seniors across the country manage inflammation and embrace a healthier, plant-based lifestyle.

Harold's kitchen, once a place of solitude and discomfort, had transformed into a hub of joy, community, and healing. As he continued to savor the flavors of his vegan anti-inflammatory diet, Harold cherished each day, grateful for the unexpected chapter of vibrancy and well-being that unfolded in his golden years.

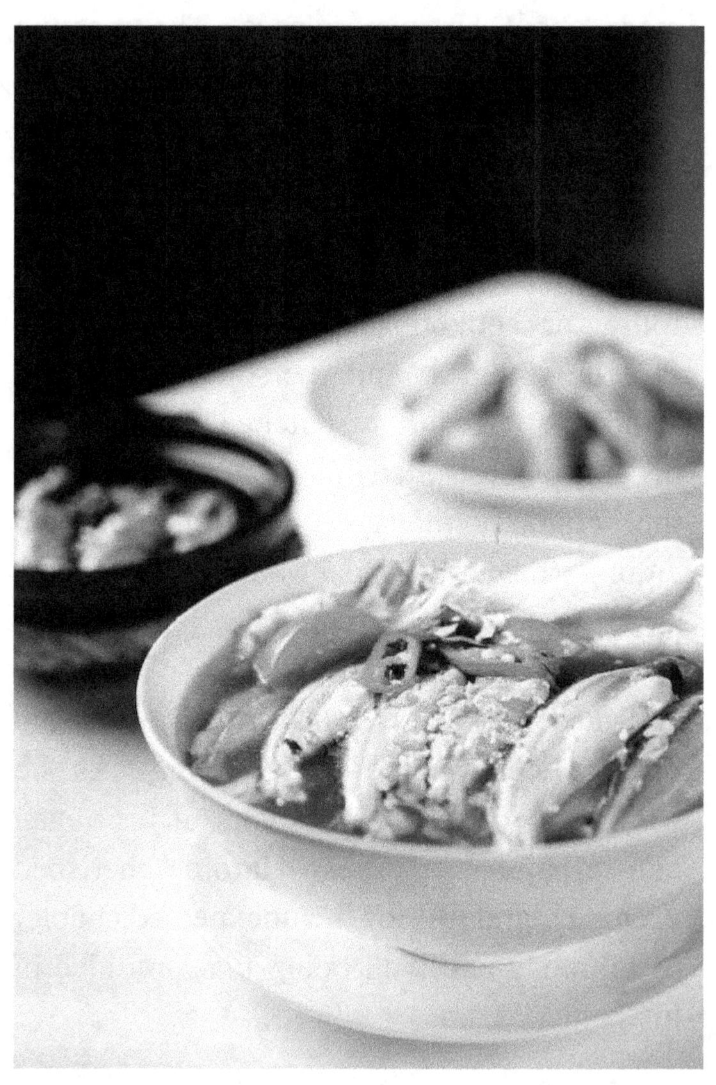

CHAPTER 1: WHAT IS ANTI-INFLAMMATORY DIET

An anti-inflammatory diet is a nutritional approach that focuses on reducing inflammation in the body, a common factor in many chronic diseases and conditions. In the context of seniors, whose bodies may be more susceptible to inflammation-related issues, adopting an anti-inflammatory diet becomes particularly important for promoting overall health and well-being. A Vegan Anti-Inflammatory Diet, as outlined in a specialized cookbook for seniors, emphasizes plant-based foods to harness the power of nature in combating inflammation.

The core principle of an anti-inflammatory diet involves incorporating foods with anti-inflammatory properties while minimizing those that contribute to inflammation. In the vegan context, this means relying on a variety of fruits, vegetables, whole grains, legumes, nuts, and seeds. These plant-based foods are rich in antioxidants, vitamins, and minerals, known for their ability to quell inflammation and support the body's immune system.

In the Vegan Anti-Inflammatory Diet Cookbook For Seniors, recipes are carefully crafted to include ingredients that not only satisfy taste buds but also provide essential nutrients to combat inflammation. Leafy greens like kale and spinach, berries bursting with antioxidants, and omega-3 fatty acid-rich seeds such as flaxseeds and chia seeds take center stage. These ingredients are known to have anti-inflammatory effects, helping to alleviate the chronic low-grade inflammation often associated with aging.

Crucially, the cookbook encourages seniors to limit or avoid processed foods, refined sugars, and saturated fats – common culprits that can trigger inflammation. By steering clear of these inflammatory triggers, seniors can further support their bodies in maintaining optimal health.

The cookbook also offers practical tips for meal planning, grocery shopping, and preparing simple yet flavorful plant-based meals. Seniors can find inspiration in diverse recipes, from hearty lentil stews to colorful vegetable stir-fries and nutrient-packed smoothies. The emphasis is not only on the health benefits but also on the pleasure of eating, ensuring that seniors can enjoy delicious and satisfying meals while prioritizing their well-being.

Vegan Anti-Inflammatory Diet, as detailed in a dedicated cookbook for seniors, provides a comprehensive and accessible guide to managing inflammation through plant-based nutrition. By incorporating a variety of wholesome ingredients and minimizing inflammatory triggers, seniors can embark on a flavorful journey toward better health and an enhanced quality of life.

EFFECT OF THE INFLAMMATION ON THE BODY

Inflammation is a natural and necessary process in the body's immune response to injury or infection. It is a complex biological response that involves the activation of immune cells, blood vessels, and molecular mediators to eliminate the cause of cell injury, clear out damaged cells, and initiate tissue repair. This acute inflammation is typically a protective and localized response.

However, chronic or prolonged inflammation can have detrimental effects on the body. It is associated with a variety of health conditions and diseases. Some of the effects of chronic inflammation include:

1. Cellular Damage: Prolonged inflammation can lead to damage of healthy cells, tissues, and organs. The constant activation of immune cells and the release of inflammatory mediators can harm surrounding structures.

2. Chronic Diseases: Chronic inflammation is linked to the development of several chronic diseases, including cardiovascular diseases, diabetes, autoimmune disorders, and neurodegenerative conditions such as Alzheimer's disease.

3. Weakened Immune System: Chronic inflammation can compromise the immune system's ability to function optimally. This may lead to an increased susceptibility to infections and other illnesses.

4. Pain and Discomfort: Inflammatory processes often lead to pain and discomfort. Conditions like arthritis, for example, involve inflammation of the joints, causing pain, swelling, and reduced mobility.

5. Increased Risk of Cancer: Persistent inflammation is associated with an increased risk of certain types of cancer. The inflammatory microenvironment can contribute to the initiation, promotion, and progression of cancer cells.

6. Contributor to Aging: Chronic inflammation has been implicated in the aging process. It can accelerate the wear and tear on the body's cells and tissues, potentially leading to premature aging.

7. Metabolic Effects: Chronic inflammation is linked to insulin resistance and metabolic syndrome, contributing to the development of type 2 diabetes and obesity.

8. Cardiovascular Effects: Inflammation plays a role in the development of atherosclerosis, a condition where arteries become narrowed and hardened due to the buildup of plaque. This can increase the risk of heart attacks and strokes.

DISEASES RELATED TO INFLAMMATION

Chronic inflammation is associated with a wide range of diseases and conditions. While inflammation is a natural and necessary response to injury or infection, persistent or inappropriate inflammation can contribute to the development and progression of various health issues.

Some of the diseases related to inflammation include:

1. Arthritis: Inflammatory joint diseases, such as rheumatoid arthritis and psoriatic arthritis, involve chronic inflammation of the joints, leading to pain, swelling, and stiffness.

2. Cardiovascular Diseases: Chronic inflammation is linked to atherosclerosis, a condition characterized by the buildup of plaque in the arteries. This can contribute to heart disease, heart attacks, and strokes.

3. Inflammatory Bowel Diseases (IBD): Conditions like Crohn's disease and ulcerative colitis involve chronic inflammation of the digestive tract, leading to symptoms such as abdominal pain, diarrhea, and weight loss.

4. Type 2 Diabetes: Inflammation is associated with insulin resistance, a key factor in the development of type 2 diabetes. Chronic inflammation can impair the body's ability to regulate blood sugar levels.

5. Neurodegenerative Diseases: Chronic inflammation has been implicated in the development and progression of neurodegenerative conditions such as Alzheimer's disease, Parkinson's disease, and multiple sclerosis.

6. Allergies: Inflammatory responses play a role in allergic reactions, causing symptoms such as itching, swelling, and respiratory issues.

7. Chronic Obstructive Pulmonary Disease (COPD): Conditions like chronic bronchitis and emphysema involve chronic inflammation of the airways, leading to breathing difficulties.

8. Autoimmune Diseases: Conditions where the immune system mistakenly attacks the body's own tissues, such as lupus, multiple sclerosis, and certain thyroid disorders, involve chronic inflammation.

9. Cancer: Chronic inflammation in the microenvironment of tissues can contribute to the initiation, promotion, and progression of cancer cells.

10. Psoriasis: This autoimmune skin condition is characterized by red, scaly patches on the skin, resulting from inflammation.

11. Periodontal Disease: Inflammation of the gums and tissues supporting the teeth can lead to periodontal disease, which is associated with conditions like gingivitis and periodontitis.

CHAPTER 2: BENEFITS OF ANTI-INFLAMMATORY DIET

Following an anti-inflammatory diet can offer a variety of health benefits, as it focuses on incorporating foods that help reduce inflammation and avoiding those that may contribute to it.

Here are core benefits of adopting an anti-inflammatory diet:

1. Reduced Chronic Inflammation: The primary goal of an anti-inflammatory diet is to reduce chronic inflammation in the body. This can help alleviate symptoms associated with various inflammatory conditions and may contribute to the prevention of chronic diseases.

2. Improved Joint Health: For individuals with arthritis or other inflammatory joint conditions, an anti-inflammatory diet can help reduce pain, swelling, and stiffness, improving overall joint health and mobility.

3. Heart Health: By promoting the consumption of heart-healthy foods and reducing inflammatory triggers, an anti-inflammatory diet can contribute to cardiovascular health. It may help lower the risk of heart disease, reduce cholesterol levels, and maintain healthy blood pressure.

4. Balanced Blood Sugar Levels: An anti-inflammatory diet, particularly one that includes whole grains, fruits, vegetables, and lean proteins, can help regulate blood sugar levels. This is beneficial for individuals with or at risk of type 2 diabetes.

5. Weight Management: Many components of an anti-inflammatory diet, such as fiber-rich fruits and vegetables, can support weight management. Maintaining a healthy weight is crucial for overall well-being and can help reduce inflammation.

6. Improved Digestive Health: An anti-inflammatory diet, especially one rich in fiber and nutrients, can promote a healthy digestive system. It may help prevent or alleviate symptoms of digestive disorders like irritable bowel syndrome (IBS) and inflammatory bowel diseases (IBD).

7. Enhanced Immune Function: The nutrients found in anti-inflammatory foods, such as antioxidants, vitamins, and minerals, support a strong immune system. This can help the body fight off infections and illnesses.

8. Better Mental Health: Some studies suggest a connection between inflammation and mental health conditions like depression. An anti-inflammatory diet, rich in omega-3 fatty acids and other nutrients, may positively influence mood and cognitive function.

9. Cancer Prevention: While not a guarantee, reducing chronic inflammation through diet may contribute to a lower risk of certain cancers. Antioxidants found in fruits and vegetables have been associated with protective effects against cancer.

10. Improved Skin Health: Certain skin conditions, like acne and psoriasis, are influenced by inflammation. A diet rich in anti-inflammatory foods may contribute to healthier skin by reducing inflammation and supporting overall skin health.

CHAPTER 3: TIPS TO ACHIEVE OPTIMAL HEALTH WITH ANTI-INFLAMMATORY DIET

Adopting an anti-inflammatory diet, especially through a Vegan Anti-Inflammatory Diet Cookbook designed for seniors, is a powerful way to promote optimum health. This plant-based approach focuses on incorporating foods with anti-inflammatory properties while avoiding those that may contribute to inflammation. Let's explore the key foods to eat and avoid to achieve optimal health in the context of this specialized cookbook.

Foods to Eat

1. Fruits and Vegetables: The foundation of a vegan anti-inflammatory diet is built on a colorful array of fruits and vegetables. These foods are rich in antioxidants, vitamins, and minerals that help combat inflammation. Berries, leafy greens, cruciferous vegetables, and citrus fruits are particularly beneficial.

2. Whole Grains: Incorporating whole grains like quinoa, brown rice, oats, and barley provides fiber and essential nutrients. These grains have a lower glycemic index, helping regulate blood sugar levels and reduce inflammation.

3. Legumes: Beans, lentils, and chickpeas are excellent sources of plant-based protein, fiber, and various anti-inflammatory compounds. They contribute to satiety and support digestive health.

4. Nuts and Seeds: Almonds, walnuts, flaxseeds, and chia seeds are packed with omega-3 fatty acids and antioxidants. These components help reduce inflammation and support heart health.

5. Healthy Fats: Include sources of healthy fats such as avocados and olive oil. These fats contain monounsaturated and polyunsaturated fats, which have anti-inflammatory effects.

6. Spices and Herbs: Turmeric, ginger, garlic, and cinnamon are known for their anti-inflammatory properties. Incorporating these spices into recipes not only enhances flavor but also boosts the anti-inflammatory benefits of meals.

7. Plant-Based Proteins: Tofu, tempeh, and other plant-based protein sources are essential for seniors to maintain muscle mass and overall health. These foods offer a wealth of nutrients without the inflammatory effects often associated with animal-based proteins.

8. Green Tea: Rich in antioxidants, green tea has anti-inflammatory and potential protective effects against chronic diseases. It serves as a hydrating and health-promoting beverage.

Foods to Avoid

1. Processed Foods: Minimize or eliminate processed foods, as they often contain additives, preservatives, and trans fats that can contribute to inflammation. This includes packaged snacks, sugary treats, and certain convenience foods.

2. Refined Sugars: High intake of refined sugars, commonly found in sweets, sugary beverages, and desserts, can lead to inflammation and negatively impact overall health. Opt for natural sweeteners like maple syrup or dates when sweetness is desired.

3. Trans Fats: Avoid sources of trans fats, which are commonly found in fried foods and some commercially baked goods. These fats can contribute to inflammation and increase the risk of cardiovascular issues.

4. Excessive Omega-6 Fatty Acids: While omega-6 fatty acids are essential, an imbalance between omega-6 and omega-3 fatty acids can promote inflammation. Reduce the intake of processed oils like corn oil and soybean oil.

5. Dairy Products: Dairy can be inflammatory for some individuals. In a vegan anti-inflammatory diet, dairy is replaced with plant-based alternatives like almond milk, soy milk, or oat milk.

6. Red and Processed Meats: High consumption of red and processed meats has been associated with inflammation and various chronic diseases. In a vegan diet, these are naturally excluded, promoting a more anti-inflammatory eating pattern.

7. Gluten (if intolerant): Some individuals may have gluten intolerance or sensitivity, leading to inflammation. In such cases, opting for gluten-free grains like quinoa or brown rice can be beneficial.

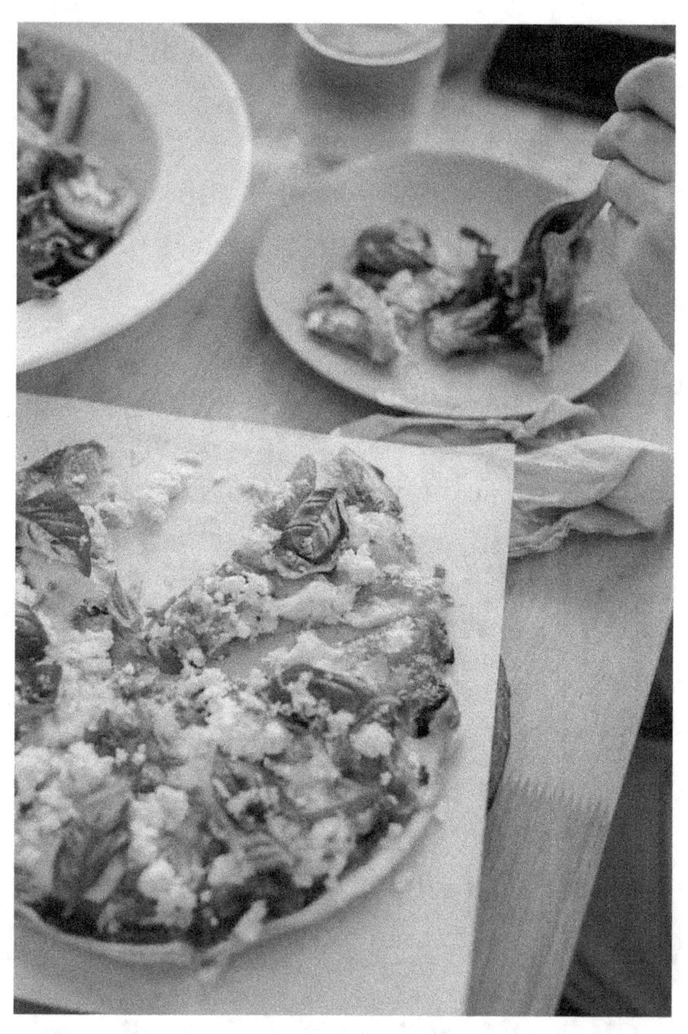

CHAPTER 4: ANTI-INFLAMMATORY RECIPES

Avocado and Chickpea Breakfast Burrito

Ingredients:
- Whole wheat tortillas (2)
- Avocado (1, mashed)
- Chickpeas (1/2 cup, cooked)
- Cherry tomatoes (1/2 cup, halved)
- Red onion (2 tbsp, finely chopped)
- Cilantro (2 tbsp, chopped)
- Lime juice (1 tbsp)
- Salt and pepper to taste

Instructions:
1. In a bowl, mash the avocado and mix it with chickpeas, cherry tomatoes, red onion, cilantro, lime juice, salt, and pepper.

2. Warm the whole wheat tortillas in a pan or microwave.
3. Spread the avocado and chickpea mixture evenly on each tortilla.
4. Roll up the tortillas into burritos and serve.

Berry Chia Seed Pudding Parfait

Ingredients:
- Chia seeds (2 tbsp)
- Almond milk (1 cup)
- Mixed berries (1/2 cup, fresh or frozen)
- Granola (1/4 cup)
- Maple syrup (1 tbsp)

Instructions:
1. Mix chia seeds and almond milk in a bowl, let it sit for 15 minutes or until it forms a gel-like consistency.
2. In a glass or bowl, layer chia pudding with mixed berries and granola.

3. Repeat the layers until the glass is filled.

4. Drizzle maple syrup on top and refrigerate for at least 2 hours or overnight.

Spinach and Tomato Tofu Scramble

Ingredients:

- Firm tofu (1/2 block, crumbled)
- Spinach (1 cup, chopped)
- Cherry tomatoes (1/2 cup, halved)
- Red onion (2 tbsp, finely chopped)
- Turmeric powder (1/2 tsp)
- Nutritional yeast (2 tbsp)
- Salt and pepper to taste

Instructions:

1. In a pan, sauté crumbled tofu with spinach, cherry tomatoes, and red onion.

2. Add turmeric powder, nutritional yeast, salt, and pepper. Cook until

spinach is wilted and tofu is heated through.

3. Serve warm as a savory breakfast scramble.

Blueberry Almond Overnight Oats

Ingredients:
- Rolled oats (1/2 cup)
- Almond milk (1/2 cup)
- Blueberries (1/4 cup, fresh or frozen)
- Almonds (2 tbsp, chopped)
- Maple syrup (1 tbsp)

Instructions:
1. In a jar, combine rolled oats, almond milk, blueberries, and chopped almonds.
2. Stir well, cover, and refrigerate overnight.
3. In the morning, drizzle with maple syrup before serving.

Sweet Potato and Black Bean Breakfast Bowl

Ingredients:

- Sweet potato (1, roasted and diced)
- Black beans (1/2 cup, cooked)
- Avocado (1/2, sliced)
- Salsa (2 tbsp)
- Fresh cilantro (2 tbsp, chopped)
- Lime wedges (for garnish)

Instructions:

1. Arrange roasted sweet potato, black beans, and avocado slices in a bowl.
2. Top with salsa and fresh cilantro.
3. Garnish with lime wedges and serve.

Quinoa and Fruit Breakfast Bowl

Ingredients:

- Quinoa (1/2 cup, cooked)
- Mixed fruit (1 cup, such as berries, kiwi, and banana)
- Almond butter (2 tbsp)
- Hemp seeds (1 tbsp)
- Coconut flakes (1 tbsp)

Instructions:

1. In a bowl, layer cooked quinoa with mixed fruit.
2. Drizzle almond butter over the top.
3. Sprinkle with hemp seeds and coconut flakes.
4. Enjoy as a refreshing and nutritious breakfast bowl.

Turmeric and Ginger Smoothie Bowl

Ingredients:

- Frozen mango chunks (1 cup)
- Banana (1, frozen)
- Almond milk (1/2 cup)
- Turmeric powder (1/2 tsp)
- Fresh ginger (1 tsp, grated)
- Toppings: granola, chia seeds, sliced kiwi

Instructions:

1. Blend frozen mango, frozen banana, almond milk, turmeric powder, and grated ginger until smooth.
2. Pour the smoothie into a bowl.
3. Top with granola, chia seeds, and sliced kiwi.

Peanut Butter and Banana Toast

Ingredients:
- Whole grain bread (2 slices, toasted)
- Peanut butter (2 tbsp)
- Banana (1, sliced)
- Cinnamon (1/2 tsp)

Instructions:
1. Spread peanut butter evenly on toasted whole grain bread slices.
2. Arrange banana slices on top.
3. Sprinkle it with cinnamon for added flavor.

Zucchini and Tomato Breakfast Hash

Ingredients:
- Zucchini (1, grated)
- Cherry tomatoes (1/2 cup, halved)
- Red bell pepper (1/4 cup, diced)

- Red onion (2 tbsp, finely chopped)
- Olive oil (1 tbsp)
- Fresh basil (2 tbsp, chopped)
- Salt and pepper to taste

Instructions:

1. In a pan, sauté grated zucchini, cherry tomatoes, red bell pepper, and red onion in olive oil.
2. Cook until vegetables are tender.
3. Season with salt and pepper, sprinkle fresh basil, and serve warm.

Chocolate Avocado Smoothie

Ingredients:

- Avocado (1/2)
- Banana (1, frozen)
- Cocoa powder (2 tbsp)
- Almond milk (1 cup)
- Maple syrup (1 tbsp, optional)
- Ice cubes (optional)

Instructions:

1. Blend avocado, frozen banana, cocoa powder, almond milk, and maple syrup until smooth.
2. Add ice cubes if desired for a colder consistency.
3. Pour into a glass and enjoy this chocolatey, nutrient-packed smoothie.

Quinoa and Vegetable Stuffed Bell Peppers

Ingredients:
- Bell peppers (2, halved)
- Quinoa (1 cup, cooked)
- Black beans (1/2 cup, cooked)
- Corn kernels (1/2 cup)
- Cherry tomatoes (1/2 cup, diced)
- Red onion (2 tbsp, finely chopped)
- Cumin (1 tsp)
- Paprika (1/2 tsp)
- Avocado (1, sliced)
- Fresh cilantro (2 tbsp, chopped)
- Lime wedges for serving

Instructions:
1. Preheat the oven to 375°F (190°C).
2. In a bowl, mix cooked quinoa, black beans, corn, cherry tomatoes, red onion, cumin, and paprika.
3. Stuff bell pepper halves with the quinoa mixture.

4. Bake for 25-30 minutes or until peppers are tender.
5. Top with avocado slices, fresh cilantro, and serve with lime wedges.

Lentil and Vegetable Curry

Ingredients:

- Lentils (1 cup, cooked)
- Cauliflower florets (1 cup)
- Carrots (1/2 cup, sliced)
- Spinach (2 cups)
- Coconut milk (1 cup)
- Curry powder (1 tbsp)
- Turmeric (1/2 tsp)
- Cumin (1 tsp)
- Garlic (2 cloves, minced)
- Ginger (1 tbsp, grated)
- Basmati rice for serving

Instructions:

1. In a pot, combine lentils, cauliflower, carrots, spinach, coconut milk, curry

powder, turmeric, cumin, garlic, and ginger.

2. Simmer until vegetables are tender.

3. Serve over cooked basmati rice.

Chickpea and Kale Salad

Ingredients:

- Chickpeas (1 can, drained and rinsed)
- Kale (2 cups, chopped)
- Cherry tomatoes (1 cup, halved)
- Cucumber (1/2, diced)
- Red bell pepper (1/2, diced)
- Kalamata olives (1/4 cup, sliced)
- Red onion (2 tbsp, finely chopped)
- Tahini dressing (3 tbsp)
- Lemon juice (1 tbsp)
- Salt and pepper to taste

Instructions:

1. In a large bowl, combine chickpeas, kale, cherry tomatoes, cucumber, red bell pepper, olives, and red onion.

2. Drizzle with tahini dressing and lemon juice.

3. Toss well and season with salt and pepper.

Sweet Potato and Lentil Buddha Bowl

Ingredients:

- Sweet potatoes (2, diced)
- Lentils (1 cup, cooked)
- Broccoli florets (1 cup)
- Red cabbage (1 cup, shredded)
- Avocado (1/2, sliced)
- Hemp seeds (2 tbsp)
- Lemon-tahini dressing (3 tbsp)
- Quinoa or brown rice for serving

Instructions:

1. Roast sweet potatoes, lentils, and broccoli in the oven until tender.

2. Assemble bowls with quinoa or brown rice, roasted vegetables, red cabbage, avocado, and hemp seeds.

3. Drizzle with lemon-tahini dressing before serving.

Mediterranean Chickpea Salad

Ingredients:

- Chickpeas (1 can, drained and rinsed)
- Cucumber (1, diced)
- Cherry tomatoes (1 cup, halved)
- Red bell pepper (1, diced)
- Kalamata olives (1/4 cup, sliced)
- Red onion (2 tbsp, finely chopped)
- Fresh parsley (2 tbsp, chopped)
- Extra virgin olive oil (2 tbsp)
- Lemon juice (1 tbsp)
- Dried oregano (1 tsp)
- Salt and pepper to taste

Instructions:

1. In a bowl, combine chickpeas, cucumber, cherry tomatoes, red bell pepper, olives, red onion, and parsley.
2. Drizzle with olive oil and lemon juice.

3. Sprinkle with dried oregano, salt, and
   pepper. Toss well before serving.

Teriyaki Tofu Stir-Fry

Ingredients:
- Firm tofu (1/2 block, cubed)
- Broccoli florets (1 cup)
- Bell peppers (1 cup, sliced)
- Carrots (1/2 cup, julienned)
- Snow peas (1/2 cup)
- Teriyaki sauce (3 tbsp)
- Sesame oil (1 tbsp)
- Garlic (2 cloves, minced)
- Ginger (1 tbsp, grated)
- Brown rice or quinoa for serving

Instructions:
1. In a wok or pan, sauté cubed tofu in
   sesame oil until golden.
2. Add broccoli, bell peppers, carrots,
   snow peas, garlic, and ginger.
3. Pour in teriyaki sauce and stir-fry
   until vegetables are tender.

4. Serve over cooked brown rice or quinoa.

Roasted Vegetable Wrap

Ingredients:
- Whole wheat wraps (2)
- Eggplant (1/2, sliced)
- Zucchini (1/2, sliced)
- Red onion (1/2, sliced)
- Hummus (1/4 cup)
- Spinach leaves (1 cup)
- Cherry tomatoes (1/2 cup, halved)
- Balsamic glaze for drizzling

Instructions:
1. Roast eggplant, zucchini, and red onion in the oven until tender.
2. Spread hummus on each wrap.
3. Layer with roasted vegetables, spinach leaves, and cherry tomatoes.
4. Drizzle with balsamic glaze, roll up, and enjoy.

Cauliflower and Chickpea Tacos

Ingredients:
- Cauliflower florets (2 cups)
- Chickpeas (1 can, drained and rinsed)
- Taco seasoning (2 tbsp)
- Corn tortillas (4)
- Avocado (1, sliced)
- Cilantro (2 tbsp, chopped)
- Lime wedges for serving

Instructions:
1. Roast cauliflower and chickpeas with taco seasoning until golden.
2. Warm corn tortillas.
3. Fill each tortilla with roasted cauliflower, chickpeas, avocado slices, and cilantro.
4. Serve with lime wedges.

Butternut Squash and Kale Risotto

Ingredients:
- Butternut squash (1 cup, diced)
- Arborio rice (1 cup)
- Vegetable broth (4 cups, heated)
- Kale (2 cups, chopped)
- Shallots (2, finely chopped)
- Garlic (2 cloves, minced)
- Nutritional yeast (2 tbsp)
- White wine (1/4 cup, optional)
- Olive oil (2 tbsp)
- Salt and pepper to taste

Instructions:
1. In a pan, sauté shallots and garlic in olive oil until softened.
2. Add Arborio rice and stir to coat in the oil.
3. If using, pour in white wine and cook until mostly absorbed.
4. Begin adding vegetable broth gradually while stirring continuously until rice is cooked.

5. In the last few minutes, stir in diced butternut squash and chopped kale.
6. Finish with nutritional yeast, salt, and pepper.

Lentil and Vegetable Stew

Ingredients:

- Lentils (1 cup, cooked)
- Carrots (2, chopped)
- Celery (2 stalks, chopped)
- Onion (1, diced)
- Garlic (3 cloves, minced)
- Tomatoes (1 can, diced)
- Vegetable broth (4 cups)
- Cumin (1 tsp)
- Paprika (1 tsp)
- Bay leaves (2)
- Salt and pepper to taste

Instructions:

1. In a large pot, sauté onions and garlic until fragrant.
2. Add carrots, celery, lentils, diced tomatoes, vegetable broth, cumin, paprika, bay leaves, salt, and pepper.

3. Simmer until vegetables and lentils are tender. Remove bay leaves before serving.

Chickpea and Spinach Curry

Ingredients:

- Chickpeas (1 can, drained and rinsed)
- Spinach (4 cups, fresh or frozen)
- Coconut milk (1 can)
- Onion (1, diced)
- Ginger (1 tbsp, minced)
- Garlic (3 cloves, minced)
- Curry powder (2 tbsp)
- Turmeric (1 tsp)
- Cayenne pepper (1/4 tsp, optional)
- Salt and pepper to taste

Instructions:

1. In a pan, sauté onions, garlic, and ginger until softened.
2. Add chickpeas, spinach, coconut milk, curry powder, turmeric, cayenne pepper, salt, and pepper.

3. Simmer until spinach wilts and flavors meld. Serve over rice or quinoa.

Quinoa-Stuffed Bell Peppers

Ingredients:
- Bell peppers (4, halved and seeds removed)
- Quinoa (1 cup, cooked)
- Black beans (1/2 cup, cooked)
- Corn kernels (1/2 cup)
- Salsa (1/2 cup)
- Cumin (1 tsp)
- Chili powder (1 tsp)
- Avocado (1, sliced)
- Fresh cilantro (2 tbsp, chopped)

Instructions:
1. Preheat the oven to 375°F (190°C).
2. In a bowl, mix quinoa, black beans, corn, salsa, cumin, and chili powder.
3. Stuff each bell pepper half with the quinoa mixture.

4. Bake for 25-30 minutes until peppers are tender.

5. Top with sliced avocado and fresh cilantro before serving.

Eggplant and Chickpea Tagine

Ingredients:

- Eggplant (1, cubed)
- Chickpeas (1 can, drained and rinsed)
- Tomatoes (2, diced)
- Onion (1, diced)
- Garlic (3 cloves, minced)
- Vegetable broth (1 cup)
- Cumin (1 tsp)
- Coriander (1 tsp)
- Smoked paprika (1 tsp)
- Cinnamon (1/2 tsp)
- Lemon zest (1 tsp)
- Fresh parsley (2 tbsp, chopped)

Instructions:

1. In a pot, sauté onions and garlic until softened.

2. Add eggplant, chickpeas, tomatoes, vegetable broth, cumin, coriander, smoked paprika, cinnamon, and lemon zest.
3. Simmer until the eggplant is tender. Garnish with fresh parsley before serving.

Butternut Squash and Coconut Curry

Ingredients:
- Butternut squash (1, peeled and cubed)
- Coconut milk (1 can)
- Red curry paste (2 tbsp)
- Onion (1, sliced)
- Ginger (1 tbsp, minced)
- Garlic (3 cloves, minced)
- Red bell pepper (1, sliced)
- Tofu (1/2 block, cubed)
- Fresh cilantro (2 tbsp, chopped)

Instructions:

1. In a pan, sauté onions, garlic, and ginger until fragrant.
2. Add butternut squash, red curry paste, coconut milk, red bell pepper, and tofu.
3. Simmer until butternut squash is tender. Garnish with fresh cilantro before serving.

Mediterranean Quinoa Salad

Ingredients:

- Quinoa (1 cup, cooked)
- Cherry tomatoes (1 cup, halved)
- Cucumber (1, diced)
- Kalamata olives (1/2 cup, sliced)
- Red onion (1/4 cup, finely chopped)
- Chickpeas (1/2 cup, cooked)
- Fresh parsley (2 tbsp, chopped)
- Lemon juice (2 tbsp)
- Olive oil (2 tbsp)
- Salt and pepper to taste

Instructions:

1. In a bowl, combine quinoa, cherry tomatoes, cucumber, olives, red onion, and chickpeas.
2. In a separate bowl, whisk together lemon juice, olive oil, salt, and pepper.
3. Pour the dressing over the salad, toss well, and garnish with fresh parsley.

Vegan Buddha Bowl

Ingredients:

- Brown rice (1 cup, cooked)
- Roasted sweet potatoes (1 cup, cubed)
- Steamed broccoli (1 cup)
- Avocado (1/2, sliced)
- Radishes (1/4 cup, sliced)
- Hummus (1/4 cup)
- Pumpkin seeds (2 tbsp)
- Tahini dressing (2 tbsp)

Instructions:

1. Arrange cooked brown rice, roasted sweet potatoes, steamed broccoli, avocado, and radishes in a bowl.
2. Add dollops of hummus and sprinkle pumpkin seeds.
3. Drizzle with tahini dressing before serving.

Vegan Lentil and Vegetable Stir-Fry

Ingredients:

- Lentils (1 cup, cooked)
- Mixed vegetables (2 cups, such as bell peppers, broccoli, and snap peas)
- Garlic (3 cloves, minced)
- Ginger (1 tbsp, minced)
- Soy sauce (2 tbsp)
- Sesame oil (1 tbsp)
- Rice vinegar (1 tbsp)
- Sriracha (1 tsp, optional)
- Green onions (2 tbsp, chopped)

Instructions:

1. In a wok or pan, sauté garlic and ginger until fragrant.
2. Add mixed vegetables and cooked lentils.
3. Stir in soy sauce, sesame oil, rice vinegar, and sriracha if using.
4. Cook until vegetables are tender. Garnish with chopped green onions.

Spaghetti Aglio e Olio with Roasted Vegetables

Ingredients:
- Whole wheat spaghetti (8 oz, cooked)
- Cherry tomatoes (1 cup, halved)
- Zucchini (1, sliced)
- Garlic (4 cloves, sliced)
- Red pepper flakes (1/2 tsp)
- Olive oil (3 tbsp)
- Fresh basil (2 tbsp, chopped)
- Salt and pepper to taste

Instructions:

1. Preheat the oven to 400°F (200°C).
2. Toss cherry tomatoes, zucchini, and sliced garlic with olive oil, salt, and pepper.
3. Roast in the oven for 15-20 minutes.
4. In a pan, sauté red pepper flakes in olive oil.
5. Toss cooked spaghetti with roasted vegetables, olive oil, and fresh basil.

Chocolate Avocado Mousse

Ingredients:
- Avocado (2, ripe)
- Cocoa powder (1/4 cup)
- Maple syrup (1/4 cup)
- Vanilla extract (1 tsp)
- Almond milk (1/4 cup)

Instructions:
1. Blend avocados, cocoa powder, maple syrup, vanilla extract, and almond milk until smooth.
2. Refrigerate for at least 2 hours before serving.

Vegan Berry Parfait

Ingredients:
- Mixed berries (1 cup)
- Coconut yogurt (1 cup)
- Granola (1/2 cup)
- Maple syrup (2 tbsp)

Instructions:

1. In a glass, layer coconut yogurt with mixed berries and granola.
2. Drizzle with maple syrup and serve.

Peanut Butter Banana Ice Cream

Ingredients:

- Bananas (4, frozen)
- Peanut butter (2 tbsp)
- Almond milk (1/4 cup)
- Dark chocolate chips (2 tbsp)

Instructions:

1. Blend frozen bananas, peanut butter, and almond milk until creamy.
2. Fold in dark chocolate chips.
3. Freeze for an additional 1-2 hours before serving.

Coconut Bliss Balls

Ingredients:

- Medjool dates (1 cup, pitted)
- Almonds (1/2 cup)
- Shredded coconut (1/4 cup)
- Cocoa powder (2 tbsp)
- Vanilla extract (1 tsp)

Instructions:

1. Blend dates, almonds, shredded coconut, cocoa powder, and vanilla extract in a food processor.
2. Roll the mixture into small balls and refrigerate for 30 minutes.

Mango Sorbet

Ingredients:

- Mango (2 cups, frozen)
- Lime juice (1 tbsp)
- Agave syrup (2 tbsp)
- Fresh mint leaves (for garnish)

Instructions:

1. Blend frozen mango, lime juice, and agave syrup until smooth.
2. Freeze for an additional 1-2 hours.
3. Garnish with fresh mint leaves before serving.

Oatmeal Raisin Cookies

Ingredients:

- Rolled oats (1 cup)
- Raisins (1/2 cup)
- Almond butter (1/2 cup)
- Maple syrup (1/4 cup)
- Cinnamon (1 tsp)

Instructions:

1. Preheat the oven to 350°F (175°C).
2. Mix rolled oats, raisins, almond butter, maple syrup, and cinnamon in a bowl.
3. Scoop spoonfuls of the mixture onto a baking sheet and bake for 12-15 minutes.

Vegan Chocolate Chip Banana Bread

Ingredients:
- Ripe bananas (3)
- Flour (2 cups)
- Baking powder (1 tsp)
- Baking soda (1/2 tsp)
- Vegan chocolate chips (1/2 cup)
- Maple syrup (1/2 cup)
- Coconut oil (1/4 cup, melted)

Instructions:
1. Preheat the oven to 350°F (175°C).
2. Mash ripe bananas and mix with flour, baking powder, baking soda, chocolate chips, maple syrup, and melted coconut oil.
3. Pour the batter into a greased loaf pan and bake for 50-60 minutes.

Raspberry Chia Seed Pudding

Ingredients:

- Chia seeds (1/4 cup)
- Almond milk (1 cup)
- Raspberry compote (1/2 cup)
- Agave syrup (2 tbsp)

Instructions:

1. Mix chia seeds and almond milk, let it sit for 15 minutes.
2. In a glass, layer chia pudding with raspberry compote.
3. Drizzle with agave syrup and refrigerate for at least 2 hours.

Almond Butter Energy Bites

Ingredients:

- Rolled oats (1 cup)
- Almond butter (1/2 cup)
- Flaxseeds (2 tbsp)
- Coconut flakes (1/4 cup)
- Maple syrup (1/4 cup)

Instructions:

1. Combine rolled oats, almond butter, flaxseeds, coconut flakes, and maple syrup in a bowl.
2. Roll the mixture into bite-sized balls and refrigerate for 30 minutes.

Apple Cinnamon Baked Oatmeal

Ingredients:

- Rolled oats (2 cups)
- Almond milk (1 1/2 cups)
- Apples (2, diced)
- Maple syrup (1/4 cup)
- Cinnamon (1 tsp)

Instructions:

1. Preheat the oven to 350°F (175°C).
2. Mix rolled oats, almond milk, diced apples, maple syrup, and cinnamon in a baking dish.
3. Bake for 30-35 minutes or until the top is golden brown.

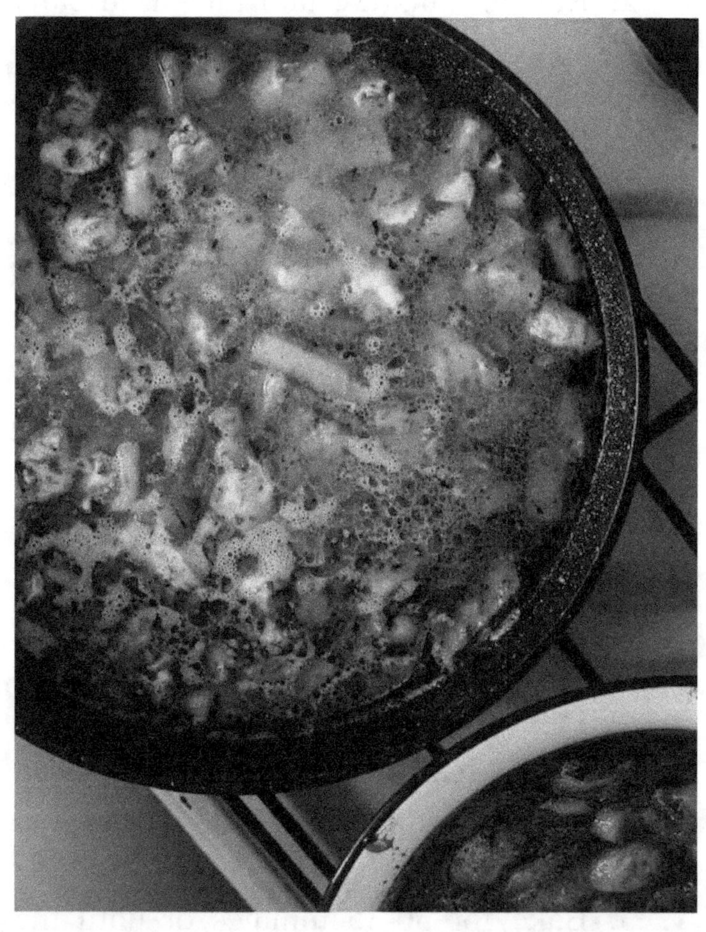

CHAPTER 5: MEAL PLANNING

HOW TO USE THE MEAL PLAN

Step 1: Review the Meal Plan:
Take a few minutes to review the 14-day vegan anti-inflammatory meal plan. Familiarize yourself with the breakfast, lunch, and dinner options for each day.

Step 2: Create a Shopping List:
Based on the meal plan, create a shopping list of the ingredients needed for the recipes. Check your pantry and fridge to see which items you already have. This ensures you have everything on hand for the upcoming week.

Step 3: Meal Prep and Batch Cooking:
Consider doing some meal prep and batch cooking to save time during the week. Prepare ingredients that can be used in

multiple recipes, such as chopping vegetables, cooking grains, or making sauces and dressings. Store these in containers for easy access.

Step 4: Follow Daily Meal Schedule:
Each day, follow the designated meal schedule. Start your day with the specified breakfast, enjoy the recommended lunch, and wrap up the day with the suggested dinner. Feel free to adjust portion sizes based on your hunger levels and personal preferences.

Step 5: Listen to Your Body and Stay Hydrated:
Pay attention to how your body responds to the meal plan. If you find yourself feeling more energized or notice improvements in digestion, that's a positive sign. Stay hydrated by drinking water throughout the day, and consider incorporating herbal teas or infused water for added variety.

14-DAY MEAL PLAN

Day 1:

Breakfast: Avocado and Chickpea Breakfast
Burrito
Lunch: Mediterranean Stuffed Acorn Squash
Dinner: Vegan Berry Parfait

Day 2:

Breakfast: Blueberry Almond Overnight
Oats
Lunch: Spinach and Tomato Tofu Scramble
Dinner: Sweet Potato and Black Bean
Breakfast Bowl

Day 3:

Breakfast: Quinoa and Fruit Breakfast Bowl
Lunch: Zucchini and Tomato Breakfast Hash
Dinner: Coconut Bliss Balls

Day 4:

Breakfast: Turmeric and Ginger Smoothie Bowl
Lunch: Peanut Butter Banana Ice Cream
Dinner: Oatmeal Raisin Cookies

Day 5:

Breakfast: Chocolate Avocado Smoothie
Lunch: Berry Chia Seed Pudding Parfait
Dinner: Vegan Chocolate Chip Banana Bread

Day 6:

Breakfast: Mango Sorbet
Lunch: Raspberry Chia Seed Pudding
Dinner: Almond Butter Energy Bites

Day 7:

Breakfast: Apple Cinnamon Baked Oatmeal
Lunch: Avocado and Chickpea Breakfast Burrito
Dinner: Mediterranean Stuffed Acorn Squash

Day 8:

Breakfast: Blueberry Almond Overnight Oats
Lunch: Spinach and Tomato Tofu Scramble
Dinner: Sweet Potato and Black Bean Breakfast Bowl

Day 9:

Breakfast: Quinoa and Fruit Breakfast Bowl
Lunch: Zucchini and Tomato Breakfast Hash
Dinner: Coconut Bliss Balls

Day 10:

Breakfast: Turmeric and Ginger Smoothie
Bowl
Lunch: Peanut Butter Banana Ice Cream
Dinner: Oatmeal Raisin Cookies

Day 11:

Breakfast: Chocolate Avocado Smoothie
Lunch: Berry Chia Seed Pudding Parfait
Dinner: Vegan Chocolate Chip Banana
Bread

Day 12:

Breakfast: Mango Sorbet
Lunch: Raspberry Chia Seed Pudding
Dinner: Almond Butter Energy Bites

Day 13:

Breakfast: Apple Cinnamon Baked Oatmeal

Lunch: Avocado and Chickpea Breakfast Burrito

Dinner: Mediterranean Stuffed Acorn Squash

Day 14:

Breakfast: Blueberry Almond Overnight Oats

Lunch: Spinach and Tomato Tofu Scramble

Dinner: Sweet Potato and Black Bean Breakfast Bowl

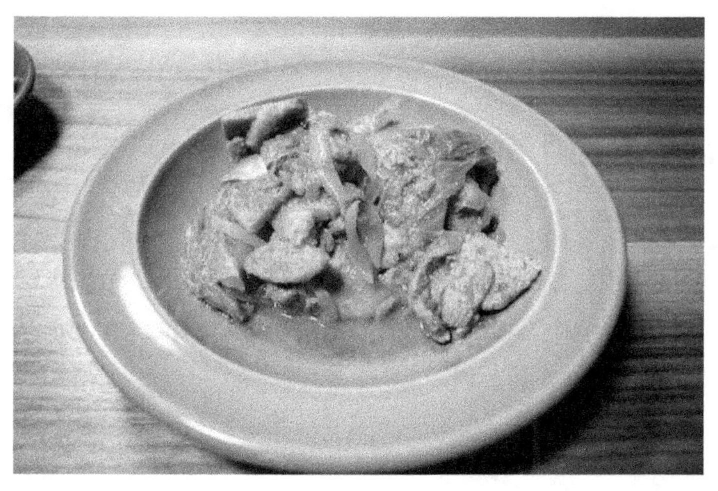

CONCLUSION

In conclusion, the Vegan Anti-Inflammatory Diet Cookbook for Seniors offers a flavorful and nutritionally rich approach to supporting overall health and well-being. By emphasizing plant-based ingredients known for their anti-inflammatory properties, the cookbook provides a diverse range of recipes tailored to the needs of seniors. From Mediterranean Stuffed Acorn Squash to Chocolate Avocado Mousse, each dish not only satisfies the taste buds but also contributes to managing inflammation associated with aging. The carefully curated meal plan promotes heart health, joint function, and immune support.

As you embark on this journey, remember that adopting and adapting to this nourishing lifestyle is a powerful choice for enhancing your quality of life. Embrace the joy of flavorful, plant-based meals and the potential benefits they bring, fostering a healthier and more vibrant senior chapter. Your well-being is the greatest motivation for this culinary adventure—nourish your body, delight your palate, and thrive in the golden years.

Thank you for choosing our Vegan Anti-Inflammatory Diet Cookbook for Seniors. We appreciate your trust in our recipes. If you enjoyed the book, please share your feedback. Your insights help us continually improve and support your wellness journey.

BONUS: WEEKLY MEAL PLANNER JOURNAL

MEAL PLANNER

Weekly

WEEK __________________ MONTH __________________

MONDAY

TUESDAY

WEDNESDAY

THURSDAY

FRIDAY

SATURDAY

SUNDAY

SHOPPING LIST

- ○ __________________
- ○ __________________
- ○ __________________
- ○ __________________
- ○ __________________
- ○ __________________
- ○ __________________
- ○ __________________
- ○ __________________
- ○ __________________
- ○ __________________
- ○ __________________
- ○ __________________

MEAL PLANNER

Weekly

WEEK ______________________   MONTH ______________________

MONDAY

SATURDAY

TUESDAY

SUNDAY

WEDNESDAY

SHOPPING LIST

THURSDAY

FRIDAY

MEAL PLANNER

Weekly

WEEK _______________   MONTH _______________

MONDAY

SATURDAY

TUESDAY

SUNDAY

WEDNESDAY

THURSDAY

FRIDAY

SHOPPING LIST

MEAL PLANNER

Weekly

WEEK ___________________   MONTH ___________________

MONDAY

TUESDAY

WEDNESDAY

THURSDAY

FRIDAY

SATURDAY

SUNDAY

SHOPPING LIST

MEAL PLANNER

Weekly

WEEK _______________________   MONTH _______________________

MONDAY

SATURDAY

TUESDAY

SUNDAY

WEDNESDAY

SHOPPING LIST

THURSDAY

FRIDAY

MEAL PLANNER

Weekly

WEEK ______________________   MONTH ______________________

MONDAY

TUESDAY

WEDNESDAY

THURSDAY

FRIDAY

SATURDAY

SUNDAY

SHOPPING LIST

MEAL PLANNER

Weekly

WEEK _________________   MONTH _________________

MONDAY

TUESDAY

WEDNESDAY

THURSDAY

FRIDAY

SATURDAY

SUNDAY

SHOPPING LIST

- ○
- ○
- ○
- ○
- ○
- ○
- ○
- ○
- ○
- ○
- ○
- ○
- ○

MEAL PLANNER

Weekly

WEEK __________________

MONTH __________________

MONDAY

TUESDAY

WEDNESDAY

THURSDAY

FRIDAY

SATURDAY

SUNDAY

SHOPPING LIST

MEAL PLANNER

Weekly

WEEK

MONTH

MONDAY

TUESDAY

WEDNESDAY

THURSDAY

FRIDAY

SATURDAY

SUNDAY

SHOPPING LIST

MEAL PLANNER

Weekly

WEEK ______________________ MONTH ______________________

MONDAY

TUESDAY

WEDNESDAY

THURSDAY

FRIDAY

SATURDAY

SUNDAY

SHOPPING LIST